I0698288

How to Cure Erectile Dysfunction without Drugs

The Absolute Guide on How to Cure ED

[RS Johnson]

Copyright © 2012 **RS Johnson**

All rights reserved.

Table of Contents

Introduction

Every year, more than 30 million men have erectile dysfunction (ED), also known as impotence; however, only about 200,000 seek medical attention. Because most men do not discuss sexual problems with their doctors, impotence remains largely undiagnosed. Furthermore, many physicians do not ask or are uncomfortable discussing the subject. ED is properly defined as the inability to maintain an erection long enough to perform intercourse and ejaculation.

While almost all men will face sexual difficulties at some point in their lives, only those unable to have successful intercourse 75 percent of the time are considered impotent. Age, contrary to popular belief, is not an unavoidable cause of impotence. It does take older men longer to develop an erection, and the force of ejaculation is reduced. Conventional medicine typically treats ED problems by prescribing a drug regimen or performing surgery. Unless low testosterone levels cause the condition, oral medications such as Erecaid or testosterone are rarely effective. Viagra, Cialis, and Levitra, which relax the corpus cavernosal smooth muscle and facilitate erections, are not without side effects. Penile injections of Papaverine or Prostaglandin E1, which affect penile blood flow, can cause prolonged erections, necessitating additional drug therapy to counteract its effects.

Furthermore, the therapy can result in penis burning and eventual fibrosis. Finally, in severe cases requiring surgical implantation, malleable or inflatable prostheses are used. Such prostheses are frequently reimplanted surgically, are uncomfortable, and fail regularly. Primary and secondary impotence can be distinguished in ED. Primary causes are uncommon, but they may be linked to low androgen levels, genetic defects, and severe psychopathology. Secondary impotence is much more common and, as the name suggests, is caused by something else, such as diabetes, arteriosclerosis, neurological disorders, psychological issues, prolonged stress, or previous genital surgery. Blood pressure and antidepressant medications can also cause impotence, especially in the elderly.

Dietary factors, which are largely ignored by conventional medicine, also contribute to the problem. Men who consume a lot of caffeine, sugar, and alcohol and men who smoke and use recreational drugs have a great risk of developing ED. However, the majority of impotence complaints are due to psychological factors. During an interview, a skilled and sensitive physician may often uncover this and suggest corrective measures.

Chapter 1| Causes, Symptoms, and Treatment of Erectile Dysfunction

Problems with any of the following systems can impair normal erectile function:

- nerve supply
- blood flow
- hormones

Physical causes

It is good to see a doctor if you have persistent erection problems because a serious medical condition could cause them. Whether the cause is minor or severe, a proper diagnosis can aid in treating any underlying medical issues and the resolution of sexual difficulties.

Poor blood flow is frequently caused by atherosclerosis. Atherosclerosis causes the arteries in the penis to narrow or clog, preventing the necessary blood flow to the penis from producing an erection.

Psychological causes

In rare cases, a man may have always had ED and never achieved an erection. If there is no physiological issue, this is referred to as primary ED, and the cause is almost always psychological. These are some examples of psychological factors:

- guilt
- Depression
- fear of intimacy
- severe anxiety

Most ED cases are classified as 'secondary.' This means that erectile function was previously normal but has become problematic. The most common causes of a new and persistent problem are physical.

Less frequently, psychological factors cause or contribute to ED, with factors ranging from treatable mental health illnesses to common emotional states that most people experience at some point in their lives.

It is important to note that medical and psychosocial causes can coexist. For example, if a man is obese, changes in blood flow can impair his ability to maintain an erection, and it is a physical cause. He may, however, have low self-esteem, which can affect erectile function and is a psychosocial cause.

Does riding a bicycle cause ED?

There are still a few questions unanswered regarding the health benefits of cycling for men.

According to some research, men who cycle for long periods may be at great risk of ED, in addition to other men's health issues like infertility and prostate cancer.

The most recent study to look into this found no link between biking and ED, but it did find a link between long hours of cycling and a higher risk of prostate cancer.

Prostate disease and ED

ED is not caused by prostate cancer. Prostate surgery to remove cancer and radiation therapy to treat prostate cancer, on the other hand, can cause ED. The condition can also be caused by the treatment of non-cancerous, benign prostate disease.

Symptoms

Men may not always achieve an erection, and if this occurs only infrequently, it is not considered a medical problem. On the other hand, ED does not only refer to an inability to achieve an erect penis.

Symptoms may also include difficulty maintaining an erection long enough to complete intercourse or an inability to ejaculate.

Emotional symptoms such as shame, anxiety, embarrassment, and a loss of interest in sexual intercourse are common.

When these symptoms occur regularly, a man is said to have ED.

Treatment of Erectile Dysfunction

The excellent thing is that there are various ED treatments available, and most men will find one that works for them properly. Among the treatments are:

Side-effects associated with PDE-5 inhibitors include:

- flushing
- visual abnormalities
- hearing loss
- indigestion
- headache

Prostaglandin E1 is a less commonly used drug option administered locally by either injecting it into the penis or properly inserting it down the urethral opening. Because most men prefer pills, these locally acting drugs are typically reserved for men who cannot take oral treatment.

Surgical treatments

There are several surgical treatment options available:

Penile implants are the last resort for men who have had no success with drug treatments or other noninvasive options.

Vascular surgery: Vascular surgery, which attempts to correct some blood vessel causes of ED, is another surgical option for some men.

Surgery is a last resort and will be used only in the most severe cases. The recovery time varies, but the success rate is high.

The primary goal of a patient's ED management strategy is to determine the etiology of the disease and treat it when possible, rather than treating the symptom alone. Modifiable or reversible factors, such as lifestyle or drug-related factors, may be associated with ED. These factors can be altered before or during the administration of specific therapies. ED can be successfully treated with current treatment options, but it cannot be cured in most cases. Only psychogenic ED, post-traumatic arteriogenic ED in young patients, and hormonal causes (e.g., hypogonadism, hyperprolactinemia) can potentially be cured with specific treatment are exceptions. Most men with ED will be treated with non-cause-specific treatment options. As a result, a structured treatment strategy is developed based on efficacy, safety, invasiveness, cost, and patient preference. To properly counsel patients in the ED, physicians must be fully informed of all treatment options. The effects of treatment options on patient and partner satisfaction and other QoL factors and efficacy and safety must be considered when evaluating treatment options.

Lifestyle Management in Erectile Dysfunction with Concomitant Risk Factors

The patient's basic workup must identify reversible risk factors for ED. Lifestyle changes and risk factor reduction must come before or after ED treatment. Individuals with ED and specific comorbid cardiovascular or metabolic diseases, such as diabetes or hypertension, may benefit the most from lifestyle changes. Aside from improving erectile function, aggressive lifestyle changes may improve overall cardiovascular and metabolic health, with recent research supporting the potential of lifestyle intervention to benefit both ED and overall health. Although more research is properly needed to determine the role of lifestyle changes in managing ED and related cardiovascular disease, they can be recommended alone or in conjunction with Phosphodiesterase (PDE5) therapy.

Some studies have suggested that when other comorbidities or risk factors are aggressively managed, the therapeutic effects of PDE5 inhibitors may be enhanced. These research results, however, have yet to be confirmed in well-controlled, long-term studies. In addition, because of the success of pharmacological therapy for ED, clinicians must provide specific evidence for the benefits of lifestyle change, which hopefully will be demonstrated in future research.

Erectile dysfunction (ED), also known as impotence, is a major issue for many men today, regardless of age — young, middle-aged, or old. Because erectile dysfunction can be caused by various factors, including a medical condition, emotional or relationship issues, certain medications, smoking, drugs, or alcohol, an erectile dysfunction cure is possible.

Though ED medication and surgery are options for treating erectile dysfunction, noninvasive erectile dysfunction remedies may benefit.

According to the Mayo Clinic, men with erectile dysfunction may experience some or all of the following persistent symptoms:

- Trouble getting an erection
- Reduced sexual desire
- Trouble keeping an erection

Erectile dysfunction medication is one of the most common reasons that young men visit their doctor. Men with erectile dysfunction frequently have diabetes or heart disease or may be sedentary or obese, but they are unaware of the impact these health conditions have on sexual function. Therefore, in addition to erectile dysfunction treatment, the doctor may advise managing the illness, increasing physical activity, or losing weight.

In addition, medication for medical conditions and alcohol and smoking can cause erectile dysfunction.

Erectile dysfunction, on the other hand, can be caused by mental health issues such as anxiety, depression, stress, and relationship issues. So it is because it is critical to seek medical attention for erectile dysfunction treatment.

If erectile dysfunction is ignored, it can lead to unsatisfactory sex life, low self-esteem, high anxiety, and relationship problems. In addition, getting a partner pregnant becomes more difficult if a man has erectile dysfunction.

Research published in The International of Sexual Medicine in May 2014 discovered that healthy lifestyle changes, including exercise, weight loss, a varied diet, and adequate sleep, could help some men reverse erectile dysfunction. The Australian researchers also demonstrated that, even if erectile dysfunction medication is required, it is more likely to be effective if these healthy lifestyle changes are implemented.

Many newer erectile dysfunction treatments can help you get a firm enough erection to have sex, and the majority have few side effects for men looking for ED medication.

Among the most commonly prescribed erectile dysfunction treatments are:

- Stendra (avanafil)
- Cialis (tadalafil)
- Viagra (sildenafil)
- Levitra or Staxyn (vardenafil)

Consult your doctor right away if you need erectile dysfunction treatment.

Chapter 2 | Natural Ways to Cure Erectile Dysfunction

Exercise Is an Active Erectile Dysfunction Treatment

"There are various lifestyle factors that can help with erectile dysfunction, but exercise is the most effective ED treatment," says Zachary R. Mucher, MD, a urologist in Sugar Land, Texas. "Exercise combats the development of ED on multiple fronts and can help reverse it once it has become a problem."

Exercise boosts blood flow, which is necessary for a strong erection, and lowers heart rate in blood vessels, which he claims is how Viagra works. In addition, weight-bearing exercise can boost testosterone production, which is important for erectile strength and sex drive.

Kegel Exercises

Kegels aren't just for women. Men can join in on the fun! Regularly performing Kegel exercises will strengthen your pelvic floor and may improve ED as well as sexual performance. The exercises are simple, and you can find instructions online or ask your doctor for more information. The standard procedure is to tighten the muscles at the bottom of your pelvic area, hold for 3 seconds, and then relax. Do this 10-15 times a day, three times a day, for optimal sexual fitness.

Everyday Exercise

Traditional exercise is also beneficial. Aerobic exercise is important for keeping your cardiovascular system in shape because arousal necessitates adequate blood flow. Maintaining a healthy weight is also an important factor in reversing erectile dysfunction. According to studies, men with a waist measurement of 42 inches or greater have a 50% greater chance of developing ED. So grab your companion and go for a long walk!

A healthy diet became one Erectile Dysfunction Treatment.

According to Dr. Mucher, the foods you eat can have a direct impact on erectile dysfunction. For example, a diet high in fruits,
A healthy diet also benefits men in maintaining a healthy body weight, which is important even though men with a 42-inch waist are 55% more likely to have ED than men with a 32-inch waist. Obesity also increases the risk of vascular disease and diabetes, both of which contribute to ED.

Sleep Is a Natural Erectile Dysfunction Treatment

Poor sleep patterns, according to Mucher, can lead to erectile dysfunction. One analysis published in the journal Brain Research highlighted the complicated link between sex hormone levels, sexual function, and sleep, finding that testosterone levels rise with improved sleep and decline with sexual dysfunction. The body's internal clock governs hormone secretion, and sleep patterns most likely help the body determine when to release specific hormones.

Maintaining a consistent sleep schedule is a natural erectile dysfunction remedy that can help ensure that those signals are clear and consistent.

Quit Smoking to Stop Erectile Dysfunction

For many men, quitting smoking is an erectile dysfunction treatment, especially if the ED is caused by vascular disease, which occurs when blood supply to the penis is restricted due to artery blockage or narrowing. Smoking and smokeless tobacco can cause the narrowing of vital blood vessels and have the same negative impact.

If you smoke, consult your doctor about quitting and whether prescription medications can help you. Smoking is bad for your heart and contributes to vascular disease, affecting blood flow to vital areas such as the genitals. To properly get maximum blood flow in all the right places, you must stop using any type of tobacco. Quitting smoking may make you more appealing in the bedroom if your partner is a nonsmoker. If your spouse smokes, you may work together to quit.

Limit Alcohol to Improve ED

Mucher warns that "alcohol is a depressant and can cause both temporary and long-term erectile dysfunction."

The central nervous system is in charge of releasing nitric oxide, which is required for the production and maintenance of an erection, and heavy alcohol consumption depresses the central nervous system, causing it to function less efficiently. A lack of nitric oxide causes erectile dysfunction. One drink may help you loosen up and get in the mood, but if you have erectile dysfunction, too much alcohol can quickly dampen your spirits. Alcohol can make your central nervous system and sexual reflexes dull. Furthermore, long-term alcohol use can damage the liver, leading to increased estrogen production in men. Drinking less can increase your enjoyment in the bedroom.

Monitor Your Meds to End Erectile Dysfunction

Erectile dysfunction can properly occur as a side effect of another health condition's medication. For example, high blood pressure medications, antidepressants, diuretics, beta-blockers, heart medications, cholesterol medications, antipsychotic drugs, hormone drugs, chemotherapy, corticosteroids, and medication for male pattern baldness are all common culprits.

If you suspect that your medication is causing ED, consult your doctor before discontinuing use. Some medicines must be weaned off with the help of a doctor.

Acupuncture May Help With Erectile Dysfunction

Although research on the efficacy of acupuncture as an erectile dysfunction treatment is conflicting, one study properly published in the Journal of Alternative and Acupuncture may be beneficial for men experiencing erectile dysfunction as a side effect of antidepressants such as selective serotonin reuptake inhibitors and serotonin noradrenaline reuptake inhibitors (SNRIs), according to a study published in Complementary Medicine in November 2013. (SNRIs).

Sexual side effects of these drugs affect at least half of all users, with some estimates putting the figure as high as 90%.

Erectile Dysfunction: Can Herbal Remedies Help or Hurt?

"Many herbal remedies claim to improve erectile function, but most have little effect and may even have harmful side effects," Mucher says. Red ginseng and pomegranate juice are two natural erectile dysfunction treatments that have shown promise.

"Ginseng is thought to properly increase nitric oxide production, which leads to improved blood flow," he explains. "Pomegranate juice is a strong antioxidant that can aid in the prevention of atherosclerosis." Always consult your doctor before taking any supplements, as they may interact with other medications you are taking.

Perk up without pills

Erectile dysfunction, known as impotence, is when a man cannot achieve or maintain an erection during sexual activity. This issue affects nearly 30 million men in the United States and can be caused by physical and psychological factors. Numerous medications are properly available to treat erectile dysfunction (ED), but many men prefer to go the natural route. Fortunately, there are several innovative approaches to tackling this problem that is low-cost and requires minimal effort.

Ginseng

Ginseng has been dubbed the "herbal Viagra," and studies have shown that taking 600-1000 milligrams three times a day can effectively treat erectile dysfunction. Make sure to get "red ginseng," a steamed and dried form of the root. If you're currently taking medication for ED or another condition, consult your doctor first to ensure there aren't any negative drug interactions.

Although Korean red ginseng has long been used to improve male sexual function, few studies have confirmed its effectiveness. In one 2002 study of 45 men with significant ED, the herb relieved symptoms of erectile dysfunction and brought "enhanced penile tip rigidity." Red ginseng is thought to promote nitric oxide synthesis, but experts aren't sure how it works. "I would recommend ginseng [for men suffering from ED]," Espinosa says. Before taking it, consult your doctor because ginseng can interact with medications you are already taking and cause allergic reactions.

L-arginine

The amino acid L-arginine is naturally present in the body and aids in producing nitric oxide, which relaxes blood vessels and causes an erection. For ED patients, as little as 5 grams of L-arginine per day can make a significant difference. Although it appears to lower blood pressure, you should consult your doctor before starting an L-arginine regimen to ensure that it does not interfere with other medications or conditions.

Watermelon

Once again, amino acids come to the rescue! For example, Citrulline, an amino acid abundant in watermelon, appears to increase blood flow to the penis. According to one study, men who took a citrulline supplement noticed an improvement in their erections and felt more satisfied. So, at the very least, incorporating watermelon into your diet means you'll be eating healthier.

Sensate Focus

Men who have erectile dysfunction for psychological reasons often respond well to techniques that involve sensory experiences rather than performance. Sensate focus exercises require a gradual build-up over several sessions to help you learn more about your own and your partner's bodies. It is excellent for reducing anxiety and establishing new patterns of expectation. More information on how to properly practice sensate focus exercises can be obtained from your doctor or therapist.

Good Conversation

Talking to your partner is one of the best natural sex tips for dealing with erectile dysfunction. A candid conversation with your partner can reduce anxiety and create a supportive environment to experiment with different treatments. When you're not in the bedroom, it's sometimes best to have sex conversations. Be aware of your body's changes and remember that physical intimacy and love are more than just sexual performance. Honesty and teamwork are frequently the natural wonders that alleviate erectile dysfunction.

Acupuncture

Though acupuncture has been properly used to treat male sexual problems for centuries, scientific evidence to support its use for erectile dysfunction is ambiguous at best. South, A systematic review of studies on acupuncture for ED was conducted by Korean researchers in 2009. Unfortunately, the researchers concluded that "the evidence is insufficient to properly suggest that acupuncture is an effective intervention for treating ED" because all of the studies had major flaws in their design.

Arginine

The amino acid L-arginine, which properly occurs naturally in food, increases the body's nitric oxide production. This compound aids erections by dilatation of blood vessels and increased blood flow to the penis. L-effectiveness arginine's against impotence has been studied, but the results have been mixed. A 1999 study published in the online journal BJU International discovered that high doses of L-arginine could help improve sexual function but only in men who have abnormal nitric oxide metabolism, such as that seen in men with cardiovascular disease (a disease that damages blood vessels). Another study, published in the Journal of Sex and Marital Therapy in 2003, discovered that ED patients who took L-arginine in conjunction with the pine extract pycnogenol experienced significant improvements in sexual function with no side effects.

According to Geo Espinosa, ND, director of the Integrative Urological Center at NYU Langone Medical Center, arginine can benefit. However, according to Espinosa, men with known cardiovascular problems should only take it under the supervision of a doctor; L-arginine can interact with some medications.

DHEA (Dehydroepiandrosterone)

Testosterone is properly required for a healthy libido and normal sexual function, and erectile dysfunction patients with low testosterone benefit from prescription testosterone replacement therapy. Similarly, taking over-the-counter supplements containing DHEA, a hormone that the body converts to testosterone and estrogen, has been properly shown in studies to help alleviate some cases of ED. However, according to McCullough, DHEA can cause side effects such as pituitary function suppression, hair loss, and acne, and its long-term safety is unknown. As a result, many experts properly advise against using supplements.

Pomegranate juice

Pomegranate juice, which is high in antioxidants, has been linked to various medical benefits, including a greatly reduced risk of heart disease and high blood pressure. Is pomegranate juice effective in preventing ED as well? There is no proof, but the results of a 2007 study were encouraging. The authors of this relatively short timeframe called for more research, claiming that larger-scale studies could demonstrate the efficacy of pomegranate juice against erectile dysfunction. "I tell my patients to drink it," Espinosa says. "It may help with ED, and even if it does not, it has other health benefits."

Yohimbe

Before the availability of Viagra and other prescription erectile dysfunction drugs, doctors would occasionally prescribe a derivative of the herb Yohimbe to their ED patients. However, experts say the medication is ineffective and can cause jitteriness and other side effects. "It's not a great drug," McCullough says. "I also suspect that the herb isn't as potent as the pharmaceutical version." Furthermore, evidence suggests that Yohimbe is linked to high blood pressure, anxiety, headaches, and other health issues. As a result, its use is discouraged by experts.

Horny goat weed

For years, horny goat weed (Epimedium) and related herbs have been touted as treatments for sexual dysfunction. However, the main compound in horny goat weed, icariin, was discovered by Italian researchers to act similarly to drugs such as sildenafil.

Lifestyle changes can improve erectile dysfunction

Whatever erectile dysfunction treatment or treatments a man ultimately chooses (whether herbal remedies or not), experts say it's critical to eat healthily and avoid smoking and heavy drinking. Furthermore, adequate exercise, stress reduction, and sleep can help many people with erection problems. Furthermore, according to Lamm, "A partner who is loving, receptive, and responsive is a home run. After all, this is still a matter between two people."

Chapter 3 | Herbal Treatment For ED

Extracts from medicinal plants have been used to treat ED for a long time in many parts, particularly in Southwest Asia. The current review properly focuses on four botanical medicinal plants whose roots are used to improve sexual performance and treat ED:

Ginkgo biloba

Ginkgo has been used to treat erectile dysfunction, particularly in cases caused by certain antidepressant medications. It is best known as a herbal treatment for cognitive decline. However, the evidence is not very convincing. One study properly published in the Journal of Sex & Marital Therapy in 1998 discovered that it did work. However, a more rigorous study, published in Human Pharmacology in 2002, could not replicate this finding. "Ginkgo has fallen out of favor in recent years," says Ronald Tamler, MD, assistant professor of medicine and co-director of Mount Sinai Medical Center's men's health program in New York City. "That's because it's not very useful. I can properly say that I have never seen ginkgo work in my practice."

There are numerous unproven herbals, dietary supplements, and natural ED treatments. Panax, propionyl-L-carnitine, L-citrulline, Rhodiola Rosea, golden root, Indian ginseng, pomegranate, zinc supplements, and ashwagandha are some examples.

1. *Eurycoma longifolia* Jack (tongkat ali);

Pausinystalia Yohimbe (yohimbine, formerly known asCorynanthe Yohimbe), Chlorophytum borivilianum (Safed Musli), Withania somnifera (ashwagandha), and Chlorophytum borivilianum (Safed Musli).

2. *E longifolia* Jack (tongkat ali)

E longifolia is a medicinal plant native to Indonesia, Malaysia, Thailand, Vietnam, and Laos (family Simaroubaceae). The most potent herbal aphrodisiac has been discovered to be the root extract. Many alkaloids, tannins, high-molecular-weight glycoproteins, quassinoids, phenolic compounds, and mucopolysaccharides are found in Tongkat Ali extracts. Eurycomaoside, butyrolactone, eurycomalactone, eurycomanone, and parvalbumin-B are the main bioactive compounds. It is thought to be natural 'Viagra.' It boosts sexual desire while improving performance and overall well-being. Other medicinal effects, such as antipyretic, antiulcer, antimalarial, antibacterial, and anti-tumor effects, have been reported in addition to its aphrodisiac effect. A root decoction has been used as a tonic. Root extract improves sexual characteristics and performance in rodents, according to laboratory animal studies. A boar model study discovered that E longifolia root extract-treated boars increased sperm counts and semen volume; the effect was attributed to increased plasma testosterone levels.

According to reports, E longifolia extract reverses estrogen's inhibitory effects on testosterone production and spermatogenesis in rats. In addition, Zakaria et al. discovered that eurycomanone, a potential bioactive compound in E longifolia root extract, induced apoptosis in hepatocarcinoma (Hep G2) cells.

Furthermore, their findings indicated that eurycomanone was cytotoxic to Hep G2 cells but not to normal Chang's liver or WLR-68 cells. Tambi and Imran investigated the effects of a water-soluble extract of E longifolia root. Jack and colleagues discovered that the extract increased sperm volume, concentration, percent of normal sperm morphology, and sperm motility in male partners of infertile couples suffering from idiopathic infertility. In male Sprague-Dawley rats, supplementation with E longifolia increased testosterone levels and increased osteoprotegerin gene expression.

3. *C borivilianum* (Safed Musli)

C borivilianum (Liliaceae) is indigenous to India. The borivilianum root contained 12 to 17 percent saponins, 1.9 to 3.5 percent stigmasterol, 0.79 percent arabinose, 3.8 percent galactose, 0.73 percent glucose, and 0.78 percent glucose rhamnose. The recommended dose for dried root powder is 5 g, and the extract dose is 500 mg. It is used as an aphrodisiac to treat ED and to improve sperm quality and volume. In addition, it prevents premature ejaculation, boosts stamina and libido, and improves general well-being and vitality. C. borivilianum significantly increased high-density lipoprotein cholesterol levels and decreased plasma and hepatic lipid profiles in hypercholesteremic rats, according to Visavadiya and Narasimhacharya.

Furthermore, the treatments increased fecal cholesterol, sterols, and bile excretion, as well as superoxide dismutase levels. In rats, Kenjale et al. assessed the aphrodisiac and spermatogenic potential of an aqueous extract of dried roots of C borivilianum. C borivilianum was administered orally at 125 mg/kg/day and 250 mg/kg/day doses. As a control, 4 mg/kg/day of Viagra (sildenafil citrate) was given. Three hours later, sexual behavior was observed using a receptive female.

On the first, seventh, fourteenth, twenty-first, and twenty-eight days of treatment, they were paired with proestrus female rats to observe their sexual behavior. The treatment was extended for 60 days in all groups except the Viagra group for sperm count. C borivilianum had significant aphrodisiac action in rats at 125 mg/kg, as evidenced by increased libido, sexual vigor, and sexual arousal. Similarly, at the higher dose, all parameters of sexual behavior were improved, but the effect was saturated after 14 days. On day 60, the sperm count properly increased significantly in both C borivilianum-treated groups. Thus, C borivilianum extract is effective in the treatment of premature ejaculation and oligospermia.

For 28 days, streptozoticin-induced diabetic male rats were given 250 mg/kg/day and 500 mg/kg/day of C borivilianum root, which improved sperm morphology and reduced oxidative stress and free radical formation. In addition, in the presence of streptozotocin and alloxan-induced hyperglycemia, aqueous extracts of C borivilianum improved sexual performance when compared to diabetic controls.

4. *W somnifera* (ashwagandha)

W somnifera (ashwagandha), also known as winter cherry (Solanaceae), is native to Africa, the Mediterranean, India, Pakistan, Afghanistan, South Africa, Bangladesh, Egypt, Morocco, Congo, and Jordan (36). The plant's roots contain steroid alkaloids and steroidal lactones, which are the main components of ashwagandha; these compounds are known as withanolides. Within is the primary constituent of the various alkaloids. Somniferin, somniferous, alanine, pseudowithanine, tropine, pseudotropine, cuscohygrine, anserine, and anhydride are the other alkaloids.

The root contains two acyl steryl glucosides (sitoindoside VII and sitoindoside VIII). Withanolides are composed of a C28 steroidal nucleus, a C9 side chain, and six-membered lactone rings. Ashwagandha root also contains flavonoids and a variety of withanolide ingredients. It is used to treat bronchitis, asthma, ulcers, insomnia, senility, and dementia and has various medicinal applications (aphrodisiac, liver tonic, anti-inflammatory agent, astringent). Animal studies and clinical trials back up the use of ashwagandha for anxiety, cognitive and neurological disorders, inflammation, and Parkinson's disease.

It also has cryoprotective properties for patients undergoing radiation and chemotherapy and benefits for nervous exhaustion. W somnifera is used to treat chronic fatigue, dehydration, bone weakness, muscle weakness, loose teeth, impotence, premature ejaculation, debility, constipation, senility, memory loss, drug withdrawal symptoms, rheumatism, nervous exhaustion, anxiety, and arthritis pain in the knee. In addition, W somnifera extracts inhibit the transcription factor nuclear factor-kappa B (NF-B), acting as an anti-inflammatory agent. This is due to its ability to interact with IKKB, a kinase responsible for nuclear translocation of NF-B and activation of inflammatory signaling pathways.

5. ***Pausinystalia johimbe* (formerly *Corynanthe johimb*e)**

Yohimbine is the main alkaloid found in the bark of the West African evergreen P. johimbe (formerly known as C johimbe), which belongs to the Rubiaceae family. Yohimbine hydrochloride (an indole alkaloid) is the main active chemical found in P johimbe bark, and it has stimulant and aphrodisiac properties.

However, the levels of yohimbine found in P johimbe bark extract vary and are frequently very low. As a result, while P johimbe bark has traditionally been used to treat ED, there is insufficient scientific evidence to form a firm conclusion in this regard. It is a 2-receptor antagonist with no direct relationship to an erection. Instead, it acts as a stimulant for sex motivation. Yohimbine has been used to treat sexual dysfunction as both an over-the-counter dietary supplement in the form of a herbal extract and as prescription medicine in purified form.

Yohimbine 20 mg or an adjusted dose is effective in treating orgasmic dysfunction. Yohimbine has recently been linked to treatment for type 2 diabetes mellitus in animal and human models with alpha-2A adrenergic receptor gene polymorphisms. According to the Institutes Of health, the standardized form of yohimbine that is available as prescription medicine in the United States is yohimbine hydrochloride, which has been shown in human studies to be successful in the prevention of male impotence. Yohimbine hydrochloride USP is a medication used to treat erectile dysfunction. Controlled studies indicate that it is not always an effective treatment for impotence, and evidence of increased sex drive (libido) is only anecdotal. It cannot be ruled out that orally administered yohimbine may be beneficial in some ED patients.

The disparities in the available data can be attributed to differences in drug design, patient selection, and the definition of a positive response. Yohimbine has been shown to reverse sexual satiety and exhaustion in male rats and increase the volume of ejaculated sperm in dogs, with the effect lasting at least 5 hours after administration. Yohimbine has been properly shown to be effective in treating male orgasmic dysfunction, sexual side effects caused by certain antidepressants, and female hypersexual disorder.

Yohimbine has several negative side effects, including anxiety. Oral yohimbine at higher doses can cause various side effects, including rapid heart rate, high blood pressure, overstimulation, insomnia, and sleeplessness. Seizures and renal failure are two more serious side effects that may occur. Yohimbine should not be consumed by people with liver, kidney, heart disease, or psychological disorders. Yohimbine has a low therapeutic index, with a narrow range between effective and dangerous doses. GGI upset, increased blood pressure, headache, agitation, rash, tachycardia, and frequent urination are possible side effects.

Conclusion

Herbal medicines have historically been shown to cure or prevent certain ailments. However, there is very little documented data to back up the dose, side effects, efficacy, and interactions. Because the efficacy and safety of herbal remedies, unlike synthetic drugs, have not been evaluated, well-controlled and randomized studies are required to establish such products' therapeutic efficacy and safety. Side effects and interactions with prescription medications must also be determined. A variety of herbal and natural products are currently being used to treat erectile dysfunction. Natural methods of treating erectile dysfunction are healthier and less dangerous than using drugs. The number of active ingredients in herbals can vary between preparations, necessitating the standardization of herbal medicines.

Visit And Buy the Other Books of This Author

Happy Saint Patrick's Day: Saint Patrick's Day Planner/Journal with 8.5x11 inches and 100 Pages

https://www.amazon.com/dp/B09BY841SZ

St. Patrick's Day: Saint Patrick's Day Planner/Journal with 8.5x11 inches and 100 Pages

https://www.amazon.com/dp/B09BY7XWGD

Happy Easter: Easter Egg Patterns Worksheet: 8.5x11 Inches 60 Pages

https://www.amazon.com/dp/B09BT2B6F3

Easter Hunt Activity Happy Easter: Easter Hunt Activity Journal | Notebook size 8.5x11 60 Pages

https://www.amazon.com/dp/B09BY7XWKL

Easter Day Spring Writing Assignment worksheet: Easter Day Spring Writing Assignment worksheet | 8.5x11 60 Pages | Spring Worksheet

https://www.amazon.com/dp/B09BY5HNVB

Cinco De Mayo: Large Updated Organizer with Daily Spreads For 2 Months with Cover Paperback https://www.amazon.com/dp/B09BY8178L

Taking full charge of your finance: Easy Guide to Personal Finance

https://www.amazon.com/Taking-full-charge-your-finance/dp/B099C8S85Z

Sure, Steps to Wealth Creation: How to Build Wealth from Nothing

https://www.amazon.com/Sure-Steps-Wealth-Creation-Nothing/dp/B099C3GNQH

All You Need to Know About Cryptocurrency: Understanding Risk and Reward in Investing

https://www.amazon.com/Need-Know-About-Cryptocurrency-Understanding/dp/B099C3GNML

Eliminating Your Debt in 12 (x) Easy Steps and Keep Them Off: A Practical Guide to Eliminating Your Debt Forever!

https://www.amazon.com/Eliminating-Your-Debt-Easy-Steps/dp/B099BZX4FX

NLP For Beginners

https://www.amazon.com/NLP-Beginners-RS-Johnson-ebook/dp/B098JBH28Q

Credit Repair Secrets

https://www.amazon.com/Credit-Repair-Secrets-RS-Johnson/dp/B098JH79X2

<-END->

www.ingramcontent.com/pod-product-compliance
Lightning Source LLC
Chambersburg PA
CBHW051926250726
48659CB00002B/872